Small Simple Changes to Weight Loss and Weight Management

Rich Kay

i

ISBN 10: 1512019232
ISBN 13: 9781512019230

What are people saying about Rich Kay's

Small Simple Changes?

"Rich Kay's Small Simple Changes gave me the confidence and self-esteem to complete my lifetime dream and goal of doing a 5k. I started with 5 minutes of exercise a week, and felt so empowered and then I was able to do 10 then 15 and last June I did my 1st 5k! Small and steady wins the race I always say!!!"

Gail Mates, National Spokeswoman American Heart Association Go Red For Women

"Rich Kay is one of the most credible people around to give fundamental words of wisdom on how to beat obesity because he has--with Small Simple Changes! Hear him speak and read his book. He motivated himself and can motivate you, too!"

Dr. Elizabeth Berbano, MD MPH Certified, American Board of Internal Medicine, Fellow of the American College of Physicians, Certified Group Fitness Instructor, American Council on Exercise

"Wow! Rich's strategies to improve your eating habits, fitness and general positive outlook on life are easy and highly effective. Your organization will greatly benefit from personally hearing his humor and inspirational message. His book is a must read for you if you have tried everything to lose weight and keep it off. Rich changes lives."

James Malinchak, Co-Author, Chicken Soup for the COLLEGE Soul, Co-Author, Chicken Soup for the ATHLETE'S Soul, 2008-2009 GKIC Marketer of the Year www.Malinchak.com

"Rich Kay is the real thing with proven keys to success. His Small Simple Changes techniques have changed lives for the better. We have served together to attack the national problem of obesity. Rich has been a key part of our Church's as well as many others churches nationally in the Losing to Live/Bod4God Program where people have lost over 4,000 pounds using his Small Simple Changes techniques as a part of our program. Rich Kay is one of the most positive and entertaining speakers on weight loss, eating habits and weight management. He is clearly on a mission to change lives for the better."

Pastor Steve Reynolds The Anti-Fat Pastor – as seen on Fox News, Author of "Bod4God, Four Keys to a Better Body" www.Bod4God.org

"Rich Kay has made it possible to take a simple approach to a very complex problem of not only losing weight but keeping it off possible for me. I have had a weight problem for years – single mom with three kids over 200 lbs go from a size 22 to a size 2. Yes I said "2". So, for all the ladies that have tried all the programs and pills this will work for you and it will help you mold your new life style into a healthy new you. I was one of those people who had about 5 different size clothes in my closet the ups and downs are gone forever thanks to his guidance and support. Rich has a way of breaking it down to "Small Simple Changes" that truly work. I am in the best shape of my life and have never felt better. If you don't like to look in the mirror – this program is for you. I now can look in the mirror and like what I see. It takes time, and he opens your eyes to see the real GOD given you. His positive attitude and inspirational speaking is out of this world, he is the real deal – he did it and can help you reach your dream you. It's almost been three years doing "Small Simple Changes" and I'm still going strong. Thanks Rich, for all you do to help others!"
Trish, Chantilly, VA

Congratulations on your decision to invest in yourself and improve your health and your life. The best investment you can ever make is in yourself. Any information you obtain to improve your life is priceless. It is clear you have a desire to change for the better. I sincerely congratulate you on this desire. It is my desire that after you read this book, you will use it again and again to continuously improve your life and share it with others.

The book cover shows a picture of me inside my old pair of 48 inch waist trousers that stretched to 50+ inches. I am now wearing 34 inch trousers. This is over 14 inches of excess body fat lost – over a foot of fat!

CONTENTS

What are People Saying about Small Simple Changes?   i

1   Who Should Read this Book?   1

2   Before You Begin   3

3   My Story – Sound Like You?   4

4   Getting Your Head Straight – The Power of   6

    Small Simple Changes

5   The Journey Begins   8

6   My First Day   10

7   The First Week   12

8   Week Two – Week Twenty-Five   14

9   The New Beginning   90

10   A Final Thought   92

    About the Author   93

    Let's Stay in Touch   94

1

WHO SHOULD READ THIS BOOK?

Do you look in the mirror and wonder what happened to you? Is it difficult for you to tie your shoes? Do you find it difficult to do the simple things in life like taking a shower or going to the bathroom? Do you get the infamous fat cramps in your sides? Do you have a closet or boxes full of clothes that you keep thinking someday you will fit into them again, but don't have any idea of when you can put them on again? What about your sex life???

If you are sick and tired of being sick and tired of being overweight and you made a decision to finally do something about it, then this book was written especially for you.

You too can with the battle of the bulge.

Are you sick and tired of carrying that extra weight around that is weighing you down physically, emotionally and even mentally?

Are you tired of the daily difficulties those extra pounds force you to deal with on a daily basis?

Would you like to regain the shape, energy and vitality of your youth? If so, read on!

Rich Kay has been where many of you are and have been. At 277 pounds and just under six feet, he was more than 100 pounds over his ideal weight. He had difficulties bending over to tie his shoes, getting out of bed in the morning and even going to the bathroom.

Rich's turning point came when he realized he was now obese. This former military man made a decision to win the battle of the bulge. Within six months, his mission was accomplished, weighing in at 198 lbs. But he did not stop there...

Now his mission is to help others win this battle and improve their quality of life. In his book "Small Simple Changes..." Rich Kay shares the series of dozens of Small Simple Changes he took over his 24-week journey to accomplish his goal. No fad diets, no starving yourself or 2-hour gym workouts.

Read his story for yourself and learn how to follow his successful method of shedding those unwanted pounds and keeping them off!

2

BEFORE YOU BEGIN

Every book I have read or commercial I have seen about a weight loss program or product recommends you consult your doctor before starting any program. How many times have you heard that? I am a regular person. I have a day job. I commute two hours a day. I have kids, a mortgage, etc., etc. I am NOT a doctor, lawyer, nutritionist or guru. I am simply a regular person who got sick and tired of being sick and tired and made a decision one day to lose weight and feel better. So, see your doctor if you have not recently. Besides, it is a good idea to get your weight recorded in your medical record. This way, when you look back on it in a few months, you will be pleasantly surprised.

I sincerely hope and desire to share this information with as many people as possible around this great world so they may too reap the many benefits I have from losing weight.

Just feeling better, having the energy to do more and gaining more self-respect have been the main benefits I have received. I think that you can see these results in your life as well.

Enjoy the journey.

3

MY STORY – SOUND LIKE YOU?

I am just another regular guy who woke up one morning being sick and tired of being sick and tired. I am a busy guy. I work 10-14 hours a day. I commute in a car for about 2 hours a day on top of that. I have three kids and 3 grandkids. I also do volunteer work in my church and community.

I rarely exercised. I could barely tie my shoes without huffing and puffing. I had a hard time just doing the simple things in life like taking a shower, going to the bathroom and playing with my grandkids. If you are more than 20 or more pounds overweight, you know what I mean. Carrying around that extra weight really slowed me down and actually kept me from doing so many things I now enjoy.

Then one day I woke up trying to get out of bed with great discomfort and said to myself I am so sick and tired of being sick and tired and made a simple choice to change that day. I started out at 277 pounds and now weigh less than 200 pounds after only just over six months of doing simple things I will cover in this book. No, I did not run five miles a day. I did not spend two plus hours daily at the gym. I did not starve myself. I just made some small simple changes to start off with that gave me incredible energy and motivation to continue on to my goal. This has resulted in me losing OVER 75 pounds and not only have I kept it off, but also my energy level, confidence and outlook on life has increased dramatically!

4

GETTING YOUR HEAD STRAIGHT – THE POWER OF SMALL SIMPLE CHANGES

If you are still looking for the magic pill or quick fix to lose weight AND keep it off – don't bother – it is not going to happen. I know you have heard folks say that they tried it all to lose weight and keep it off, but I can certainly and honestly say I have been pretty close to trying them all. You know pills, potions, belts, tapes, videos, all kinds of little gadgets and exercise equipment, etc. Been there, done that, got the T-shirt and had a huge credit card bill as a result of it.

To lose weight AND keep it off, I believe you first have to get MAD! Yes, MAD! I mean REALLY MAD. Mad at who or what you may ask? Good question. That extra weight on you that shows as your love handles, pot belly, big butt, thighs or wherever else fat builds on your body is NOT the real you. It is the result of those simple choices you and I have made over the years.

You know, the extra scoop of ice cream, the doughnut or going back for second servings. You made small choices that put on that weight, and you CAN make simple little choices to begin to take if off and keep it off. So don't get mad at yourself, get mad at the stuff that is calling you to instantly gratify yourself, but kills you in the long run.

You know what it is. It is the extra scoop of ice cream, doughnut or those second servings you don't need. Hey, it is okay to eat some ice cream. I did as I went through my journey.

But I used some serious personal self-talk to make small simple changes to make a huge improvement in my life. You will see what I mean later in this book.

Here is what I mean. One day I TRIED to roll out of bed and felt the pain and extreme effort it took to do this simple thing and just got mad. I mean REALLY MAD. I looked at my body and had the following self-talk:

What the heck did you do to yourself Rich? This is NOT you. Look at your old pictures. Just ten years ago, you were less than 200 pounds, wore 34-inch waste jeans and felt okay to take your shirt off on the beach. Now you buy dark clothes to hide the fat rolls, your waist size now exceeds your age and you are ashamed of even thinking about going to the beach with a shirt on! It is time to change. Rome was not build in a day. You did not gain this weight overnight. You WILL lose it over time and get back to being ME!

So began the journey. I began to make small simple changes in my lifestyle that eventually led to me losing on an average of 2-4 pounds a week! Some weeks I lost up to 5 pounds, other weeks I would plateau or level off and not lose any weight. You will probably plateau as well, that is, not see any weight loss progress, but then boom, the next week 1-5 pounds will fall off again just from making Small Simple Changes. Later in this book, I will explain in detail all the Small Simple Changes I made that brought me to my goal of being less than 200 pounds from my previous 277 pounds.

5

THE JOURNEY BEGINS

Most of the remainder of this book will be written in the first person present, tense. What? Wasn't that something I missed in English/Language class? For example, I am feeling great instead of I will feel great or I want to feel great. Based on all the successful folks I have read about and talked to, this way of thinking or self-talk in our heads drives us closer and closer to our goals until we reach them. I know, it may sound strange. But think about it for a minute. Do you smile because you are happy or are you happy because you are smiling?

Hey, I don't know all the psychology behind this, but I personally know it works. So, most of this book will be written like this so as you read, you are reading and thinking in the "I" frame of reference.

So, now that you have reached deep down and got really really MAD, now it is time to focus that anger into productive energy. Remember, you did not gain all that weight overnight, so you will make small simple changes to lose it over time.

This is a journey. Your initial goal or destination is to lose the weight to get back to the real you. Once you reach that initial

destination, your journey continues. The journey is called life.
The problem with most programs is that many people reach their
goal and then go back to their old destructive habits and gain it
back. The battle of weight loss AND weight maintenance is won or
lost in your head.

It all starts there. That is why we started with getting your head
straight and getting mad. Hold onto that. All along your journey to
your initial destination of getting back to the real you, you will use
this anger to get you there. Once you reach your goal, that anger
will be replaced with great confidence and self-respect that will
keep you on track to continue the journey indefinitely.

We take journeys every day, for example, a road trip, a business
flight or a short trip to the store. On all of these journeys, we check
to ensure we are on track but begin with navigation questions in
our mind. Just as a pilot or driver constantly checks certain gauges
to check on the progress of the journey to the destination, we need
to as well on our journey.

We all do it unconsciously. We check the gas gauge to ensure we
have enough fuel. We check road signs to ensure we are on track.
So, since this weight loss destination is a journey, we too will use
gauges to measure and check our progress. While you may think
the only gauge that counts on this weight loss and weight
maintenance journey is the scale, it is not. The scale is only one of
many gauges you need to be aware of and read.

The first and by far the MOST IMPORTANT gauge is your
head – your self-talk.

The remainder of this book is written in my own self-talk, the
conversations I had with myself during this journey. The key points
to remember are you will feel like you are off course sometimes,
but like any good pilot, STOP, and think HOW can you get back
on course.

Enjoy the journey back to the real you!

6

MY FIRST DAY

I am sooooooo mad. I cannot believe I let myself go like this. Look at me. I can't even get out of bed without getting cramps. This is going to end today!

Okay, where is that yellow sticky and my pen. I write on the yellow sticky I will be 199 pounds by September 23rd and post it on the mirror in my bathroom. That's it. I will see this every time I am in the bathroom and either see it consciously or unconsciously and it will be pounded into my head.

That's what those advertisers do to keep their brand on your mind. So I will use this same idea to keep my goal in my head. What am I thinking? I am 277 pounds today. Am I kidding myself? How will I get to 199 pounds by September 23rd?

Okay Rich, you did not gain this weight overnight and you are not going to lose it overnight. You eat an elephant one bite at a time.

Okay, today I will make one small simple change-one bite of the elephant today. What will that be? I know, I will park my car further away from my job office door so I can walk just a little further each day.

But that is just one thing. I am REALLY MAD. What else can I do? Okay Rich, one bite at a time. Tomorrow I will make another small simple change.

Okay, off to work.

First Day of Small Simple Changes:

- ✓ Got Mad
- ✓ Wrote down my goal
- ✓ Made one small simple change to get to my goal – park car further away from my office door
- ✓ Beginning weight: 277 pounds

7

THE FIRST WEEK

Getting out of bed. Okay, 199 by September 23rd. What one small simple change do I do today? Hey, parking the car over a few hundred feet from the entrance to my office instead of by the door was pretty easy. Besides, it is much easier to find my car among the sea of cars when I get off at night because no one else parks in the far away spots. Hey, that was a good idea – positive reinforcement of new habit.

Now, what do I do today? Okay, so I am not exercising yet, but hey, I have not exercised in a while and I don't want to kill myself. But, hey, parking the car further away is a start. Okay Rich, one bite at a time. Bite, hmmm, okay so I made a small simple change in activity, but what about the way I eat.

What can I do that I can stick to and not get discouraged? I hate those diets--eat this, eat that, don't do this, do that, etc. I need to do something I can easily do and continue to do. Hmmm, I remember my brother Larry always has a water bottle with him. I can't believe he is still wearing the same size blue jeans he wore in high school. I know he does more than drink water to keep in shape, but hey, I will start drinking more water. I will buy a bottle and drink it before every meal. I will refill it 3-5 times daily from the water fountain at work and drink more water in between meals.

First Week of Small Simple Changes:

- ✓ Still Mad
- ✓ Drank 3-5 Bottles of Water
- ✓ Parked Car further away at work and the stores I went to
- ✓ Looked at the Yellow Sticky note of my goal 4 times
- ✓ End of week weight: 274 – lost 3 pounds!

8

WEEK TWO

Okay, making traction. Feeling better. 199 pounds by September 23rd is going to happen. Man, I lost 3 pounds last week! Now 274 pounds. Awesome! Now what about this week?

Okay, now that I am starting to move more, let's take a crack at how I eat. My brother Larry said he eats to live and I live to eat. Hmm. He is right. I really like food – all kinds. But I don't have to be a pig about it.

Why do I eat sooooo much at each meal? Then I feel like drained afterwards. I want to take a nap after I eat. I am sooo tired of those eat this/eat that diets. I know I need carbs, fats and proteins. If I cut out the fats totally, my body will just change the carbs or protein into fat because I know my body needs some fat. I just eat toooo fast. I don't give my stomach a chance to tell my brain, hey you are full, STOP.

I know what I can do this week. I will eat slower. I will take a bite and chew until the food is really mushy. I will really taste it. I will drink water before the meal. Eat slowly and drink water during the meal. Yeah, that is what I will do.

Week 2 Small Simple Changes:

- ✓ Still Mad
- ✓ Drank 3-5 Bottles of Water daily
- ✓ Parked Car further away at work and stores
- ✓ Looked at the Yellow Sticky note of my goal 4 times
- ✓ daily
- ✓ Ate slower and drank water before and during meals
- ✓ End of week weight: 271 – lost 3 pounds this week!

WEEK THREE

Wow, lost another 3 pounds. 271 pounds – YEAH! Now what about this week? What small simple change or new habit can I introduce into my day so I can stick with it. Drinking more water is really energizing me. I go to the bathroom more, but hey, I like the increased energy. Parking the car further away from places I go is really working. I also get to get some sun and check out other nice cars on my way to work or the store. Now what about this week?

Eating slowly seems to be working. I don't feel like taking a nap after I eat anymore. I noticed that when I feel full I still have food left on my plate, especially when I eat out. I realize it is okay to not finish your plate and no one in another country is going to starve if I don't finish my plate. But I hate to throw that food away. It just seems wasteful. But man, those portions when I eat out are sooooo big. Hmm, what about doggy bags?

I know, I can continue to eat slow, drink water before and after meals and save the sandwich or doggy bag to munch on in between meals. I know I read somewhere and hear many folks say we should eat 5-6 times a day. 3 meals and snacks in between. Why not use the leftovers to munch on in between the meals? Then I won't feel starved when I eat my meal. Yeah, that is it. I will do that this week.

Week 3 Small Simple Changes:

- ✓ Still Mad
- ✓ Drank 3-5 Bottles of Water daily
- ✓ Parked Car further away at work and stores
- ✓ Looked at the Yellow Sticky note of my goal 4 times daily
- ✓ Ate slower and drank water before and during meals
- ✓ Ate leftovers in between meals
- ✓ End of week weight: 267 – lost 4 pounds this week!

WEEK FOUR

Holy Mackerel! I lost 4 pounds this past week. Now I am 267. I broke through the 270's and now am in the 260's. Wow! Awesome. It looks like those small simple changes I made the first few weeks are really working! If those small simple changes did that much, I really need to think of other ones.

Now for this week. Hmm. Okay, so I have focused on living to eat instead of eating to live. Eating slowly is definitely working along with the in-between snacks of the leftovers. Drinking more water is really feeling great. At first I felt bloated. But now my body knows I am going to give it water more frequently instead of drinking like a camel and storing it up. So I don't feel bloated anymore now that my body knows more water is coming.

Since I have more energy from the small simple changes in eating, I need to focus on the activity side. I like walking more when I park far away. Now I need to hit the stairs at work. I really don't need to take the elevator to the second floor. Wow, that is lazy come to think of it.

That is what I will do this week. I will take the stairs every time I need to get to the second floor. Hey, it is not doing 40 minutes of cardio on a treadmill, but it is better than what I am doing now - nothing. Eat the elephant one bite at a time, Rich...

Week 4 Small Simple Changes:

- ✓ Still Mad
- ✓ Drank 3-5 Bottles of Water daily
- ✓ Parked Car further away at work and stores
- ✓ Looked at the Yellow Sticky note of my goal 4 times daily
- ✓ Ate slower and drank water before and during meals
- ✓ Ate leftovers in between meals
- ✓ Taking Stairs to the 2nd Floor at work
- ✓ End of week weight: 265 – lost 2 pounds this week!

WEEK FIVE

Hmm. Only lost 2 pounds this past week. Now I am 265. Okay, hey it is still a weight loss. I know it is just 2 pounds. But when I pick up a 2 pound pack of lunch meat at the supermarket, it puts it into perspective for me. That is 2 pounds of fat I no longer have on my body. I lost over 3 pounds the first couple of weeks, but only 2 last week. So, I need to introduce another small simple change AND continue to do the others ones that have brought me this far. Hey, so far I have lost 12 pounds. That is huge!

Now for this week. Eating slowly is really coming to me easy now. I need to remember to snack in between with the leftovers. I am doing really well on drinking more water. Parking further away is fun. The stair walking was tough at first, but by the end of last week I really started to not feel tired when I got to the top. I need to continue this.

Okay, so now, I will crank up the activity level. I feel like I have more energy. I don't feel bloated anymore. I don't feel tired after meals. So what else can I do this week?

I heard someone talk about green tea. Tea, hmm. Sounds natural. I will start drinking it and see if there are other ways to take it such as a pill or sprinkle it on food. I don't want to take any of those "loose a million pounds in 5 seconds" pills. I tried those before and they made my heart race and feel hyper all the time. So I will start drinking green tea.

Also, I can start looking at all "automatic" things in life and see if I can do them manual. When I was a child, there were not too many automatic door openers to stores or escalators or even a remote control for the TV. I know. I can start going manual. Hey it is not running a marathon, but every little bit counts. If I burn 5-20 calories when I open a big door or get off the couch to change the channel and do that 10 to 20 times a day, that could be over 200 calories! I remember a million years ago when I ran on the treadmill, it took me over 30 minutes of running to do that! I know calorie counting is not the total answer, but I do know, more activity means using and building your muscles and muscle burns fat better even after I finished doing something with any of my muscles.

I will think "manual" this week.

Week 5 Small Simple Changes:

- ✓ Still Mad
- ✓ Drank 3-5 Bottles of Water daily
- ✓ Parked Car further away at work and stores
- ✓ Looked at the Yellow Sticky note of my goal 4 times daily
- ✓ Ate slower and drank water before and during meals
- ✓ Ate leftovers in between meals
- ✓ Took Stairs to the 2nd Floor at work
- ✓ Drank Green Tea daily
- ✓ Went Manual
- ✓ End of week weight: 260 – lost 5 pounds this week!

WEEK SIX

Yee Haa! I lost 5 pounds. Now I am 260. That is 17 whopping pounds of lard off my body. Wow! I feel GRRRRRREAT! I am amazed at how my body works. Just only lost 2 pounds the other week and now 5 pounds. Wow. I am definitely doing something right.

I am sooooo pumped. So now what do I add this week? Introducing these small simple changes of new tiny habits are really working.

So, eating slowly is really working for me. I now remember to snack in between with the leftovers. Drinking more water is now second nature to me. Parking further away is still fun. The stair walking is coming easier. Starting to drink green tea daily is okay, but it doesn't taste that good. I need to find another flavor of green tea. Maybe I can buy a cold one in a bottle. I like iced tea, so I will look for the cold green tea. Hopefully that will taste better.

Going "manual" was sort of fun. Trying to find stuff to do manually instead of automatic was like a game this week. I actually liked pushing those doors and getting my butt off the couch to change the channel and volume. These are all good. I will continue to do these.

So for this week, I will look at eating since last week I cranked up the activity level. I definitely have more energy now and can think clearer. I seem to have the ability to focus more and not fade after 2:00 pm. So on the eating side, I think I will eat the multi-grain bread and wheat bread instead of the white bread.

I heard when white bread is made all the natural nutrients are sucked out to keep it fresh longer and artificial stuff is put in.

Wheat and multi-grain bread seem more natural and I am seeing a lot more if it in the stores. I don't need to go to an obscure health food store to buy it. I want to go to a health food store and check some stuff out, but I will do that down the road. For now, I need to keep it simple.

I also heard wheat and multi-grain bread contains a bunch of fiber and fiber helps clean your pipes and keeps the bowels moving. Since drinking more water took away the bloated feeling, maybe this new bread will work on the other set of pipes and clean me out. That is what I will try this week.

Week 6 Small Simple Changes:

- ✓ Still Mad
- ✓ Drank 3-5 Bottles of Water daily
- ✓ Parked Car further away at work and stores
- ✓ Looked at the Yellow Sticky note of my goal 4 times daily
- ✓ Ate slower and drank water before and during meals
- ✓ Ate leftovers in between meals
- ✓ Took Stairs to the 2nd Floor at work
- ✓ Drank Green Tea daily
- ✓ Went Manual
- ✓ End of week weight: 257 – lost 3 pounds this week!

WEEK SEVEN

Yee Haa! I lost 3 pounds. Now I am 257. I broke through another 10 pound barrier. I am in the 250's! Super! That is 20 pounds so far. That is what my granddaughter weighs!

I am amazed how all those small simple new habits are so automatic now. Eating slowly snacking in between with the leftovers, drinking more water, parking further away, stair walking. This new cold drink green tea is pretty good. I can see myself drinking one to two of these daily. I need to buy them by the case. Going "manual" is going great. I actually find a reason to stand up more just to get vertical from sitting or lying down. I get out of my car more often instead of before saying to myself, never mind. I will continue to do these "going more manual" things.

Eating the multi-grain bread and wheat bread instead of the white bread was interesting. On the 2nd day this week after eating I was definitely having more healthy bowel movements. I remember my father who is 84 now, saying his doc said he had the colon of a 25 year old. I know he must eat this kind of bread. It was a little uncomfortable at first. Sort of like when I started drinking more water and feeling bloated, but by the end of the week, I felt pretty good. No more straining on the stool. I will definitely keep this up. Since I worked on eating last week, let's mix it up and think about activity. I remember reading or hearing that the word "breakfast" means breaking the fast from not eating all night. I also remember someone saying breakfast was the most important meal of the day. It kicks off your metabolism. Sort of like throwing a log on the fire to get it hot again.

I also remember reading that the best time to exercise is in the morning. Realistically, I don't have time to go to a gym or spend 30-40 minutes in the morning on exercising. Hmmm, I will just eat the elephant one bite at a time or again set a realistic goal. Before I shower I will do some small, simple stuff like jumping jacks or crunches just to let my body know there is more to come.

Besides, now that I have this increased energy, I need to focus it on new positive habits. So that is what I will do, just 2-3 minutes of simple exercises. Heck, I stop and watch the news that long to watch who killed who. I will replace that with 2-3 minutes of simple exercises to light off the metabolism and get the fire going before breakfast.

Week 7 Small Simple Changes:

- ✓ Still Mad
- ✓ Drank 3-5 Bottles of Water daily
- ✓ Parked Car further away at work and stores
- ✓ Looked at the Yellow Sticky note of my goal 4 times daily
- ✓ Ate slower and drank water before and during meals
- ✓ Ate leftovers in between meals
- ✓ Took Stairs to the 2nd Floor at work
- ✓ Drank Green Tea daily
- ✓ Went Manual
- ✓ Began simple exercises when I got out of bed to get the
- ✓ metabolism going
- ✓ End of week weight: 255 – lost 2 pounds this week

WEEK EIGHT

Okay, 2 pounds of fat fell off this past week. Now I am 255. 6 pounds away from the 240 pound barrier. I would like to see more than 2 pounds, but hey, 2 pounds a week is just fine.

I feel like an airline pilot moving towards my destination. Each week I am getting closer and closer to my destination. Sure, some weeks I get more miles or lose more pounds, but the important point to remember is I AM making progress every week no matter how small or big.

All those new small simple changes are now automatic pilot habits. Positive habits. Eating slowly, snacking in between meals with the leftovers, drinking more water, parking further away, stair walking, drinking green tea, thinking more and doing more about going "manual," eating the multi-grain bread and wheat bread is feeling pretty good too.

Adding the small simple change of 2-3 minutes of exercises in the morning has really kicked my metabolism up. My energy level is increasing and my focus is improving. No more 2:00 pm'ish sluggishness.

Now back to this week and adding something new. Let's go back to eating again. Eating slowly is definitely working. Also, when I eat with company, talking to folks in between bites has helped me slow down my eating. I not only enjoy the food more but enjoy the company more as well. Drinking water is working as well. Now I need refine it a bit more. My thinking has definitely changed about not finishing my plate. I can now not feel guilty about not finishing my entire meal. I now know it is okay.

I am learning to eat with my stomach, not with my eyes. I remember reading somewhere your portion for each meal should be about the size of your palm.

I also ran into someone who mentioned we should eat meals the size of our fist since our stomach is about the size of our fist. Hmm, two sources.

I talked to a doctor that week and asked her how big is our stomach? She said about the size of your hand, but it stretches. I remember when I was a child a friend of mine told me that once he fed his dog over 3 pounds of hot dogs!

The dog just kept eating and eating he said. He then said when he stopped feeding his dog all those hotdogs, the poor dog rolled over moaning. When he felt his stomach, it was rock hard. I guess it stretched to accommodate all that food. While the dog could physically eat that much, it was definitely NOT good for him.

So, this week I will focus on portion sizes and eat meals the size of my hand. When I go to the buffet, I will resist overfilling my plate with food. It is the same price whether I get 3 pounds of food overflowing on my plate or get enough to comfortably fill my stomach which is about the size of my hand. I will continue to eat carbs, proteins and fats.

Week 8 Small Simple Changes:

- ✓ Still Mad
- ✓ Drank 3-5 Bottles of Water daily
- ✓ Parked Car further away at work and stores
- ✓ Looked at the Yellow Sticky note of my goal 4 times daily
- ✓ Ate slower and drank water before and during meals
- ✓ Ate leftovers in between meals
- ✓ Took Stairs to the 2nd Floor at work
- ✓ Drank Green Tea daily
- ✓ Went Manual
- ✓ Began simple exercises when I got out of bed to get the metabolism going
- ✓ Ate with my stomach not with my eyes - eat meals the size of your hand
- ✓ End of week weight: 252 – lost 3 pounds this week

WEEK NINE

3 pounds less this week. Now I am 252. Only 3 more pounds away from the 240's. Continuing to stay MAD at my fat, not me, but my fat is really keeping me going. Not only is staying MAD at my fat helping me, I also am feeling much better about myself. I have lost 25 pounds. 25 pounds – that is incredible! That's like carrying around a heavy car battery wrapped around you.

Auto pilot is really working now. I think about all those new small simple changes I made and how they are working. What a great idea to introduce one small simple change a week. I remember hearing that if you do something for 21 days it will more than likely become a habit. This is both for positive habits and bad habits.

Slower eating, snacking in-between meals with the leftovers, drinking 3-5 bottles of water daily, parking further away, stair walking, drinking green tea, thinking more and doing more about going "manual" and eating the multi-grain bread and wheat bread are all now part of my positive routine. I am starting to look forward to doing the 2-3 minutes of exercise when I get up. I really see the benefits of increased energy throughout the day. I think I will do a few more minutes and check out some other ones I can do at home like maybe knee push-ups, crunches and other ones in addition to jumping jacks and toe touches.

Eating with my stomach not with my eyes went pretty good this week. A few times I wanted to add more, but eating slower and drinking water definitely helped. I am still snacking in-between meals. I added apples, pears and bananas to my in between meal snacks in addition to the left-overs. Good choice. Any natural food is definitely good for me. I really enjoy the taste of them now too when I chew them slowly. I don't need sweets anymore. I lost the craving for sweets when I starting drinking more water.

Mixing it up weekly is good. I don't want to overwhelm myself and get discouraged with too many changes. Focusing on adding a new small simple change with how and what I eat one week, then focusing on adding a different activity the following week is working pretty well.

I think this week I will step up the activity a bit. Instead of going couch potato and laying on the sofa when I get home. I will take a walk around the neighborhood after I eat. I like to walk now. Those 25 extra pounds I shed over the past eight weeks really slowed me down before but now I feel pretty good.

Week 9 Small Simple Changes:

- ✓ Still Mad, but really feeling Good!
- ✓ Drank 3-5 Bottles of Water daily
- ✓ Parked Car further away at work and stores
- ✓ Looked at the Yellow Sticky note of my goal 4 times daily
- ✓ Ate slower and drank water before and during meals
- ✓ Ate leftovers in between meals
- ✓ Took Stairs to the 2nd Floor at work
- ✓ Drank Green Tea daily
- ✓ Went Manual
- ✓ Began simple exercises when I got out of bed to get the metabolism going
- ✓ Ate with my stomach not with my eyes - eat meals the size of your hand
- ✓ Took leisurely walks around the neighborhood
- ✓ End of week weight: 249.5 – lost 2.5 pounds this week

WEEK TEN

Broke the 240's pound barrier! Wooo WHOOOOO! Lost 2.5
pounds. Okay, I started measuring half pounds, but hey, it is a half
pound! Plus I am in the 240's now. Super, super, super. 249.5
pounds – getting close to losing 30 pounds so far. Feeling
Goooood.

My anger is now turning into disgust and confidence. When I see
my old picture weighing 277 pounds I feel disgusted. But I feel so
much more confident now. When people who have not seen me in
weeks see me now they say, "wow, what are you doing? You look
great!" That really feels good. But that is just little sprinkles on the
cake. What really keeps me going is seeing and recognizing MY
progress and congratulating MYSELF. Improving my self-talk with
positive language and seeing the results of the new small simple
changes is inspiring me to continue on this journey.

I introduced over 10 small simple changes since I have started and
not only have I lost close to 30 pounds, my energy level,
confidence and outlook on life is in general so much better. It is
amazing how losing weight and getting closer to the REAL you
underneath all that fat can improve things in soooo many areas of
your life.

So far slower eating, snacking in between meals with the leftovers, drinking 3-5 bottles of water daily, parking further away, stair walking, drinking green tea, thinking more about and doing more about "going manual," eating the multi-grain bread and wheat bread, 2-3 minutes of exercise when I get up, eating with my stomach not with my eyes, and starting the evening walk after eating instead of going couch potato and laying on the sofa when I get home are a whole bunch of positive new small simple changes that are having such a profound impact on me. I have to keep this going.

What to add this week? Hmmm. Last week I stepped up the activity, let's stick with what works and try something new with how or what I eat this week. The wheat and multi-grain bread are working pretty well. I have more energy and consistent bowel movements now. I heard somewhere that folks who are overweight should replace all white flour products with wheat or multi/whole grains. Since I like the taste of wheat multi-grain bread, I am going to add this new small simple change this week. Anything with white flour, pasta, crackers, etc., I will replace with a wheat or multi/whole grain version. Anything that looks like it has white flour in it I will question it and see if there is a wheat or multi/whole grain alternative.

Week 10 Small Simple Changes:

- ✓ Still Mad, but really feeling Good!
- ✓ Drank 3-5 Bottles of Water daily
- ✓ Parked Car further away at work and stores
- ✓ Looked at the Yellow Sticky note of my goal 4 times daily
- ✓ Ate slower and drank water before and during meals
- ✓ Ate leftovers in between meals
- ✓ Took Stairs to the 2nd Floor at work
- ✓ Drank Green Tea daily
- ✓ Went Manual
- ✓ Began simple exercises when I got out of bed to get the metabolism going
- ✓ Ate with my stomach not with my eyes - eat meals the size of your hand
- ✓ Took leisurely walks around the neighborhood
- ✓ Replaced all white flour products with wheat or multi/whole grains
- ✓ End of week weight: 246.5 – lost 3 pounds this week

WEEK ELEVEN

Making progress. Another 2 pounds. Steady results. Getting closer to my goal of 199 pounds. Lost over 30 pounds now. This is great.

Feeling great. Trousers getting looser. Had to tailor some trousers to fit. What a great feeling. I can't remember when I ever did that. I usually took clothes to the tailors to make them bigger...

All right, what about this week? So far I added over 10 small simple changes since I have started.

Slower eating, snacking in-between meals with the leftovers, drinking 3-5 bottles of water daily, parking further away, stair walking, drinking green tea, going "manual", eating the multigrain bread and wheat bread, 2-3 minutes of exercise when I get up, eating with my stomach not with my eyes and the evening walk after eating are really working and changing my body to the real me and giving me a more positive outlook on life. Replacing white flour products with wheat or multi-grains was pretty easy. Pasta and bagels taste pretty good in wheat flavor. That was an easy one to add.

How about this week? I really am enjoying the pump in the morning from the 2-3 minutes of exercise. But I need to spice it up a little bit. I like fast music with a beat. I know, I will play some fast moving music and crank up the simple exercises to 7- 8 minutes. I think I will start with 12 reps and 2-3 sets and work it up from there. I know my body is ready for it now.

Week 11 Small Simple Changes:

- ✓ Still Mad, but really feeling Good!
- ✓ Drank 3-5 Bottles of Water daily
- ✓ Parked Car further away at work and stores
- ✓ Looked at the Yellow Sticky note of my goal 4 times daily
- ✓ Ate slower and drank water before and during meals
- ✓ Ate leftovers in between meals
- ✓ Took Stairs to the 2nd Floor at work
- ✓ Drank Green Tea daily
- ✓ Went Manual
- ✓ Began simple exercises when I got out of bed to get the metabolism going
- ✓ Ate with my stomach not with my eyes - eat meals the size of your hand
- ✓ Took leisurely walks around the neighborhood
- ✓ Replaced all white flour products with wheat or multi/whole grains
- ✓ Added music to my morning exercises – cranked up exercises to 7-8 minutes
- ✓ End of week weight: 244.5 – lost 2 pounds this week

WEEK TWELVE

Another 2 pounds of lard off me. This is awesome. It is incredible how my body is transforming back to the real me. I have soooo much energy now.

I liked adding the music to my morning workout. It really gets me going. Those 7-8 minutes flew on by as I listened to the songs. It keeps me going to the end of each song anticipating the next up-beat song.

Okay, for this week, I think I will mix it up and add both an eating small simple change and an activity small simple change. Since I started doing crunches, my stomach area is feeling better. I can bend over more easily. I think I will increase the number of abdominal crunches each week by 10.

Now on the eating side, I need to replace my "comfort food" cravings with something a little healthier. I heard celery is a negative caloric food—that means it takes more energy to break it down than the amount of calories each little stalk is in calories. Not sure if this is true or not, but hey, I always went by the rule if it is green or natural, it must be okay for you. But celery is not exactly chocolate. I will figure out something I can put on it to spice it up like hummus or peanut butter, carbs and protein – good mix. I will continue with the slower eating, snacking in between meals with the leftovers, drinking 3-5 bottles of water daily, parking further away, stair walking, drinking green tea, going "manual," eating the multi-grain bread and wheat bread, 2-3 minutes of exercise when I get up, eating with my stomach not with my eyes, the evening walk after eating, replacing white flour products with wheat or multi-grains was pretty easy and cranking up the music along with a few more minutes of exercise in the morning.

Week 12 Small Simple Changes:

- ✓ Still Mad, but really feeling Good!
- ✓ Drank 3-5 Bottles of Water daily
- ✓ Parked Car further away at work and stores
- ✓ Looked at the Yellow Sticky note of my goal 4 times daily
- ✓ Ate slower and drank water before and during meals
- ✓ Ate leftovers in between meals
- ✓ Took Stairs to the 2nd Floor at work
- ✓ Drank Green Tea daily
- ✓ Went Manual
- ✓ Began simple exercises when I got out of bed to get the metabolism going
- ✓ Ate with my stomach not with my eyes - eat meals the size of your hand
- ✓ Took leisurely walks around the neighborhood
- ✓ Replaced all white flour products with wheat or multi/whole grains
- ✓ Added music to my morning exercises – cranked up exercises to 7-8 minutes
- ✓ Increased abdominal crunches by 10
- ✓ Replaced my "comfort food" cravings with celery and peanut butter and hummus
- ✓ End of week weight: 240 – lost 4.5 pounds this week

WEEK THIRTEEN

Wow! Lost 4.5 pounds! This is INCREDIBLE! 230's right around the corner. Lost almost 40 pounds so far and gaining momentum.

Adding the celery and cranking up the crunches plus all the other small simple changes is really having a transformational impact on me. These small simple changes are automatic to me now. I look forward to doing all these small simple things. They are now a part of me. It is effortless now.

I will continue with the slower eating, snacking in between meals with the leftovers, drinking 3-5 bottles of water daily, parking further away, stair walking, drinking green tea, going "manual," eating the multi-grain bread and wheat bread, 2-3 minutes of exercise when I get up, eating with my stomach not with my eyes, the evening walk after eating, replacing white flour products with wheat or multi-grains was pretty easy and cranking up the music along with a few more minutes of exercise in the morning. Snacking on celery with garlic hummus or peanut butter and increasing my crunches was super.

For this week I will focus on solidifying all the new small simple changes I added in the past few weeks. The earlier ones seem to come naturally. I will write these down and look at them frequently throughout the day and remind myself about them. Especially the "go manual" small simple change. I want to find more ways to increase my motion.

Week 13 Small Simple Changes:

- ✓ Still Mad, but really feeling Good!
- ✓ Drank 3-5 Bottles of Water daily
- ✓ Parked Car further away at work and stores
- ✓ Looked at the Yellow Sticky note of my goal 4 times daily
- ✓ Ate slower and drank water before and during meals
- ✓ Ate leftovers in between meals
- ✓ Took Stairs to the 2nd Floor at work
- ✓ Drank Green Tea daily
- ✓ Went Manual
- ✓ Began simple exercises when I got out of bed to get the metabolism going
- ✓ Ate with my stomach not with my eyes - eat meals the size of your hand
- ✓ Took leisurely walks around the neighborhood
- ✓ Replaced all white flour products with wheat or multi/whole grains
- ✓ Added music to my morning exercises – cranked up exercises to 7-8 minutes
- ✓ Increased crunches by 10
- ✓ Replaced my "comfort food" cravings with celery and peanut butter and hummus
- ✓ Reviewed and reinforced small simple changes
- ✓ End of week weight: 240 – did not lose any pounds this week

WEEK FOURTEEN

Hmmm. 240 again. No lost weight this week. I'm a little bit disappointed, but let's review.

I added the celery and cranked up the crunches. I continued with the slower eating, snacking in between meals with the leftovers, drinking 3-5 bottles of water daily, parking further away, stair walking, drinking green tea, going "manual," eating the multi-grain bread and wheat bread, 2-3 minutes of exercise when I get up, eating with my stomach not with my eyes, the evening walk after eating, replacing white flour products with wheat or multi-grains was pretty easy and cranking up the music along with a few more minutes of exercise in the morning.

I also focused on solidifying all the new small simple changes I added in the past few weeks. I read somewhere the body plateaus during weight loss. Okay, I will not sweat it or get depressed about it. Besides, this is the first week over the past few months that I did not drop any weight. I have lost 37 pounds so far, so what I have been doing so far has definitely worked.

I think it is time to work on the head more to get my progress going. I will dig out those old CDs and tapes I used to listen to by nationally known speakers on motivational, achievement and self-help topics and see if I can pick up some tips there. <u>I know I need to feed my mind with good stuff as much as I need to feed my body with good stuff</u>. That is what I will do this week to keep the momentum going. I will listen to positive personal and professional improvement tapes and CDs during my daily commute.

Week 14 Small Simple Changes:

- ✓ Still Mad, but really feeling Good!
- ✓ Drank 3-5 Bottles of Water daily
- ✓ Parked Car further away at work and stores
- ✓ Looked at the Yellow Sticky note of my goal 4 times daily
- ✓ Ate slower and drank water before and during meals
- ✓ Ate leftovers in between meals
- ✓ Took Stairs to the 2nd Floor at work
- ✓ Drank Green Tea daily
- ✓ Went Manual
- ✓ Began simple exercises when I got out of bed to get the metabolism going
- ✓ Ate with my stomach not with my eyes - eat meals the size of your hand
- ✓ Took leisurely walks around the neighborhood
- ✓ Replaced all white flour products with wheat or multi/whole grains
- ✓ Added music to my morning exercises – cranked up exercises to 7-8 minutes
- ✓ Increased crunches by 10
- ✓ Replaced my "comfort food" cravings with celery and peanut butter and hummus
- ✓ Reviewed and reinforced small simple changes
- ✓ Listened to positive personal and professional improvement tapes and CDs during my commute
- ✓ End of week weight: 233.5 – lost 6.5 pounds this week!!!

WEEK FIFTEEN

Holy cow! From 240 pounds to 233.5 pounds. That is 6.5 pounds in one week! Wow! That is the most I have ever lost. This is INCREDIBLE! What a major boost. I simply continued with all the small simple changes and started feeding my mind with positive personal and professional improvement information and POW – lost 6.5 pounds in one week. Wow, I guess that plateau was a short rest for my body before going down a big hill. I am soooooo pumped. I have to keep this going. I can actually see my feet when I look down without sucking in my gut.

So, let's recap. I started listening to positive personal and professional information on CDs and tapes during my commute. This is like a University on Wheels. I really picked up a bunch of good information. I love to listen to underdog stories about how regular people reach and exceed their goals.

I added the celery and cranked up the crunches. I continued with the slower eating, snacking in-between meals with the leftovers, drinking 3-5 bottles of water daily, parking further away, stair walking, drinking green tea, going "manual," eating the multi-grain bread and wheat bread, 2-3 minutes of exercise when I got up, eating with my stomach not with my eyes, the evening walk after eating, replacing white flour products with wheat or multi-grains was pretty easy and cranking up the music along with a few more minutes of exercise in the morning.

I continued to focus on solidifying all the new small simple changes I added in the past few weeks.

I keep hearing that drinking more water is good. So to remind myself to drink more water, I bought a six-pack water-carrying thingie. I fill it up in the morning before going to work and bring it home empty. I will continue to solidify this habit this week.

This is awesome!

Week 15 Small Simple Changes:

- ✓ Still Mad, but really feeling Good!
- ✓ Drank 3-5 Bottles of Water daily
- ✓ Parked Car further away at work and stores
- ✓ Looked at the Yellow Sticky note of my goal 4 times daily
- ✓ Ate slower and drank water before and during meals
- ✓ Ate leftovers and fruit in between meals
- ✓ Took Stairs to the 2nd Floor at work
- ✓ Drank Green Tea daily
- ✓ Went Manual
- ✓ Began simple exercises when I got out of bed to get the metabolism going
- ✓ Ate with my stomach not with my eyes - eat meals the size of your hand
- ✓ Took leisurely walks around the neighborhood
- ✓ Replaced all white flour products with wheat or multi/whole grains
- ✓ Added music to my morning exercises – cranked up exercises to 7-8 minutes
- ✓ Increased crunches by 10
- ✓ Replaced my "comfort food" cravings with celery and peanut butter and hummus
- ✓ Reviewed and reinforced my small simple changes
- ✓ Listened to positive personal and professional improvement tapes and CDs during my commute

- ✓ Filled up six-pack water carrying thingie with bottled water and finished each day
- ✓ End of week weight: 229.5 – lost 4 pounds this week!!!

WEEK SIXTEEN

229.5 pounds. Wow, I blasted through the 230 pound barrier in just two weeks. I had a plateau and weighed the same for two weeks. I am glad I did not give up when I did not see any weight loss for two weeks. Now, boom, blown right past the 230s. 229.5 – almost lost 40 pounds so far! I can tie my shoes with ease now and get in and out of bed easy.

Listening to positive personal and professional information on CDs and tapes during my commute is super. Eating celery and cranking up the crunches was super. I continued with the slower eating, snacking in between meals with the leftovers, drinking 5-7 bottles of water daily, parking further away, stair walking, drinking green tea, and going "manual". Still eating the multi-grain bread and wheat bread, doing the 7-9 minutes of exercises when I get up, eating with my stomach not with my eyes, still doing the evening walk after eating, replacing white flour products with wheat or multi-grains and cranking up the music with exercise in the morning.

I continued to focus on solidifying all the new small simple changes I've added in the past few weeks and drinking more water because I now use that six-pack water carrying thingie. This is all good.

For this week, as I sit in my chair at work working on the computer, I will start some leg lifts. While sitting in my chair, I will sit up straight and lift my feet off the floor for a few seconds. I will start with doing five of these 2-3 times a day while at work. I can now feel my ab muscles. Now I want to concentrate on exercising those muscles because I hear that when you exercise a certain group of muscles, they will continue to burn fat while resting! I need to do more research on that topic too.

Week 16 Small Simple Changes:

- ✓ Still Mad, but really feeling Good!
- ✓ Drank 3-5 Bottles of Water daily
- ✓ Parked Car further away at work and stores
- ✓ Looked at the Yellow Sticky note of my goal 4 times daily
- ✓ Ate slower and drank water before and during meals
- ✓ Ate leftovers and fruit in between meals
- ✓ Took Stairs to the 2nd Floor at work
- ✓ Drank Green Tea daily
- ✓ Went Manual
- ✓ Began simple exercises when I got out of bed to get the metabolism going
- ✓ Ate with my stomach not with my eyes - eat meals the size of your hand
- ✓ Took leisurely walks around the neighborhood
- ✓ Replaced all white flour products with wheat or multi/whole grains
- ✓ Added music to my morning exercises – cranked up exercises to 7-8 minutes
- ✓ Increased crunches by 10
- ✓ Replaced my "comfort food" cravings with celery and peanut butter and hummus
- ✓ Reviewed and reinforced my small simple changes
- ✓ Listened to positive personal and professional improvement tapes and CDs during my commute

- ✓ Filled up six-pack water carrying thingie with bottled water and finished each day
- ✓ Started sitting leg lifts while at work at my computer 5 reps, 2-3 times a day
- ✓ End of week weight: 225 – lost 4.5 pounds this week!!!

WEEK SEVENTEEN

Another amazing 4.5 pounds! This is super. I don't feel hungry, eating more often throughout the day and have more energy. I have lost over 50 pounds! That is more than my 5-year-old granddaughter weighs! 225 pounds now from the start of 277 pounds. These small simple changes have really had an impact. I will keep them going.

I enjoyed adding those sitting leg lifts while at work in front of my computer. It actually gave me a mental boost and a good break from what I was doing. It helped me to get recharged. I will work on keeping that one going. I like listening to positive personal and professional information on CDs and tapes during my commute. I am learning something new almost daily.

Still eating celery, doing more crunches, eating slower, snacking in between meals with the leftovers, drinking 5-7 bottles of water daily now, parking further away, stair walking, drinking green tea, going "manual" more, eating the multi-grain bread and wheat bread, doing 7-9 minutes of exercise when I get up, eating with my stomach not with my eyes, walking in the evening, replacing white flour products with wheat or multigrain and cranking up the music with exercise in the morning and using that six-pack water carrying thingie to ensure I drink 5-7 bottles of water a day.

A friend of mine, Susan, mentioned to me that she heard somewhere we should drink half our weight in ounces of water daily. So at 200+ pounds, that is 100 ounces of water. Sounds like a bunch, but using those 16 ounce bottles and drinking 6-7 of those daily, that is around 100 ounces or so.

For this week, I will continue to review and reinforce all those small simple changes, especially the one added in the past few weeks. The others are automatic now. But I will consciously think about them a few times this week to take stock in my success of adding them and sticking to them. Positive reinforcement is important. I will do some research on muscles burning fat at rest. Perhaps I will add some small weight training exercises to my morning exercises.

Week 17 Small Simple Changes:

- ✓ Still Mad, but really feeling Good!
- ✓ Drank 3-5 Bottles of Water daily
- ✓ Parked Car further away at work and stores
- ✓ Looked at the Yellow Sticky note of my goal 4 times daily
- ✓ Ate slower and drank water before and during meals
- ✓ Ate leftovers and fruit in between meals
- ✓ Took Stairs to the 2nd Floor at work
- ✓ Drank Green Tea daily
- ✓ Went Manual
- ✓ Began simple exercises when I got out of bed to get the metabolism going
- ✓ Ate with my stomach not with my eyes - eat meals the size of your hand
- ✓ Took leisurely walks around the neighborhood
- ✓ Replaced all white flour products with wheat or multi/whole grains
- ✓ Added music to my morning exercises – cranked up exercises to 7-8 minutes
- ✓ Increased crunches by 10
- ✓ Replaced my "comfort food" cravings with celery and peanut butter and hummus
- ✓ Reviewed and reinforced my small simple changes
- ✓ Listened to positive personal and professional improvement tapes and CDs during my commute

- ✓ Filled up six-pack water carrying thingie with bottled water and finished each day
- ✓ Started sitting leg lifts while at work at my computer 5 reps, 2-3 times a day
- ✓ Reviewed small simple changes and reinforced all, especially those ones added in the past few weeks
- ✓ End of week weight: 225.5 – gained weight, a half of pound????

WEEK EIGHTEEN

Gained a half pound??? Okay, no big deal. Let's review. I started out at 277 pounds. I now weigh 225.5 pounds. This is a weight loss of over 50 pounds. Over 50 pounds! I read somewhere that losing 2-3 pounds a week is about the right speed of losing weight to remain healthy and no yo-yo back to the old weight. I did not lose all this weight overnight. I had gone on a plateau once already. I zipped right past the 230 pound barrier. Having another plateau is not a bad thing.

I will continue to focus on my successes so far. I feel super. I can do so many things now I could not do before. I have more energy to play with my grandchildren. I can do the simple things in life with so much ease now. I am getting all kinds of compliments from people about my weight loss.

I will continue with sitting leg lifts while at work in front of my computer, listening to positive personal and professional information on CDs and tapes during my commute, eating celery, doing more crunches, eating slower, snacking in between meals with the leftovers, drinking 5-7 bottles of water daily now, parking further away, stair walking, drinking green tea, going "manual" more, eating the multi-grain bread and wheat bread, doing 7-9 minutes of exercise when I get up, eating with my stomach not with my eyes, walking in the evening, replacing white flour products with wheat or multigrain and cranking up the music with exercise in the morning and using that six-pack water carrying thingie to ensure I drink 5-7 bottles of water a day.

I did some reading on how our muscles burn fat at rest. Wow, that is incredible. The more muscle you have, the more fat it burns, even while at rest! While I admire and respect the achievements of bodybuilders, my goal right now is not to be a Mr. America or Mr. Universe, but I can certainly add a little muscle here and there and tone in some other places. I will get some light dumbbells and incorporate some arm, biceps and triceps weight exercises into my morning routine.

Week 18 Small Simple Changes:

- ✓ Still Mad, but really feeling Good!
- ✓ Drank 3-5 Bottles of Water daily
- ✓ Parked Car further away at work and stores
- ✓ Looked at the Yellow Sticky note of my goal 4 times daily
- ✓ Ate slower and drank water before and during meals
- ✓ Ate leftovers and fruit in between meals
- ✓ Took Stairs to the 2nd Floor at work
- ✓ Drank Green Tea daily
- ✓ Went Manual
- ✓ Began simple exercises when I got out of bed to get the metabolism going
- ✓ Ate with my stomach not with my eyes - eat meals the size of your hand
- ✓ Took leisurely walks around the neighborhood
- ✓ Replaced all white flour products with wheat or multi/whole grains
- ✓ Added music to my morning exercises – cranked up exercises to 7-8 minutes
- ✓ Increased crunches by 10
- ✓ Replaced my "comfort food" cravings with celery and peanut butter and hummus
- ✓ Reviewed and reinforced my small simple changes
- ✓ Listened to positive personal and professional improvement tapes and CDs during my commute

- ✓ Filled up six-pack water carrying thingie with bottled water and finished each day
- ✓ Started sitting leg lifts while at work at my computer 5 reps, 2-3 times a day
- ✓ Reviewed small simple changes and reinforced all, especially those ones added in the past few weeks
- ✓ Incorporated some arm, biceps and triceps weight exercises into my morning exercise routine
- ✓ End of week weight: 222 pounds – lost 3 pounds

WEEK NINETEEN

Okay then, we had a little rest on the plateau, now a loss of 3 pounds. Down to 222. Awesome.

Doing those few sets of biceps and triceps curls was fun. Those dumbbells only cost a few bucks at Walmart. I didn't need to spend a gazillion dollars on some exercise machine like I did in the past and only used it a few times before it turned into a dust collector. Hey, wait a minute. If building this little muscle gave me a breakthrough after the last plateau, I need to add some more.

I have that old abdominal machine in my basement collecting dust. Time to dust it off and incorporate it into my morning exercises. Although I am doing some crunches already, this Ab machine will work on other parts of my Abdomen and wake up some of those old out-of-shape muscles. I like that idea of muscle burning fat at rest. Okay, so for this week, I will start using that old Ab machine in the morning.

I will continue with sitting leg lifts while at work in front of my computer, listening to positive personal and professional information on CDs and tapes during my commute, eating celery, doing more crunches, eating slower, snacking in between meals with the leftovers, drinking 5-7 bottles of water daily now, parking further away, stair walking, drinking green tea, going "manual" more, eating the multi-grain bread and wheat bread, doing 7-9 minutes of exercise when I get up, eating with my stomach not with my eyes, walking in the evening, replacing white flour products with wheat or multigrain and cranking up the music with exercise in the morning and using that six-pack water carrying thingie to ensure I drink 5-7 bottles of water a day.

I will also continue with the biceps and triceps curls, but do them every other day. I remember from high school gym class the teacher said muscles need a day of rest in-between to rebuild them after being worked on.

Week 19 Small Simple Changes:

- ✓ Still Mad, but really feeling Good!
- ✓ Drank 3-5 Bottles of Water daily
- ✓ Parked Car further away at work and stores
- ✓ Looked at the Yellow Sticky note of my goal 4 times daily
- ✓ Ate slower and drank water before and during meals
- ✓ Ate leftovers and fruit in between meals
- ✓ Took Stairs to the 2nd Floor at work
- ✓ Drank Green Tea daily
- ✓ Went Manual
- ✓ Began simple exercises when I got out of bed to get the metabolism going
- ✓ Ate with my stomach not with my eyes - eat meals the size of your hand
- ✓ Took leisurely walks around the neighborhood
- ✓ Replaced all white flour products with wheat or multi/whole grains
- ✓ Added music to my morning exercises – cranked up exercises to 7-8 minutes
- ✓ Increased crunches by 10
- ✓ Replaced my "comfort food" cravings with celery and peanut butter and hummus
- ✓ Reviewed and reinforced my small simple changes
- ✓ Listened to positive personal and professional improvement tapes and CDs during my commute

- ✓ Filled up six-pack water carrying thingie with bottled water and finished each day
- ✓ Started sitting leg lifts while at work at my computer 5 reps, 2-3 times a day
- ✓ Reviewed small simple changes and reinforced all, especially those ones added in the past few weeks
- ✓ Incorporated some arm, biceps and triceps weight exercises into my morning exercise routine
- ✓ Started using that old Abdominal machine in the morning
- ✓ End of week weight: 218 pounds – lost 4 pounds

WEEK TWENTY

Cranking away. Another 4 pounds. Wow. 3 pounds the other week and now 4 pounds lost. Blasted through the 220s, now I am down to 218 pounds. I am 19 pounds away from my goal of being less than 200 pounds! I can't wait. I have to keep up this progress.

Using the old Ab machine in the morning definitely woke up some old muscles. I can feel them. I was a little sore the first day or so, but now it feels good. I think I will add another set of ab exercises at night after I get home from work. That will energize me for the rest of the night right before my evening walk.

Biceps and triceps exercises are feeling super. I am still doing sitting leg lifts while at work in front of my computer, listening to positive personal and professional information on CDs and tapes during my commute, eating celery, doing crunches on the Ab machine, eating slower, snacking in between meals with the leftovers, drinking 5-7 bottles of water daily now, parking further away, stair walking, drinking green tea, going "manual" more, eating the multi-grain bread and wheat bread, doing 7-9 minutes of exercise when I get up, eating with my stomach not with my eyes, walking in the evening, replacing white flour products with wheat or multi-grains and cranking up the music with exercise in the morning and using that six-pack water carrying thingie to ensure I drink 5-7 bottles of water a day.

Making progress. I will keep all these small simple changes that are now part of me going.

Week 20 Small Simple Changes:

- ✓ Still Mad, but really feeling Good!
- ✓ Drank 3-5 Bottles of Water daily
- ✓ Parked Car further away at work and stores
- ✓ Looked at the Yellow Sticky note of my goal 4 times daily
- ✓ Ate slower and drank water before and during meals
- ✓ Ate leftovers and fruit in between meals
- ✓ Took Stairs to the 2nd Floor at work
- ✓ Drank Green Tea daily
- ✓ Went Manual
- ✓ Began simple exercises when I got out of bed to get the metabolism going
- ✓ Ate with my stomach not with my eyes - eat meals the size of your hand
- ✓ Took leisurely walks around the neighborhood
- ✓ Replaced all white flour products with wheat or multi/whole grains
- ✓ Added music to my morning exercises – cranked up exercises to 7-8 minutes
- ✓ Increased crunches by 10
- ✓ Replaced my "comfort food" cravings with celery and peanut butter and hummus
- ✓ Reviewed and reinforced my small simple changes
- ✓ Listened to positive personal and professional improvement tapes and CDs during my commute

- ✓ Filled up six-pack water carrying thingie with bottled water and finished each day
- ✓ Started sitting leg lifts while at work at my computer 5 reps, 2-3 times a day
- ✓ Reviewed small simple changes and reinforced all, especially those ones added in the past few weeks
- ✓ Incorporated some arm, biceps and triceps weight exercises into my morning exercise routine
- ✓ Started using that old Abdominal machine in the morning
- ✓ Started using that old Abdominal machine in the evening too
- ✓ End of week weight: 214 pounds – lost 4 pounds

WEEK TWENTY-ONE

Whoooo weeee. Making major progress. 199 pounds goal in sight now. Lost another 4 pounds. 214 pounds now. 15 pounds from my goal of being less than 200 pounds. 199 pounds here I come!

Doing the old Ab machine in the morning and evening is definitely cranking up my metabolism. I feel super bending over or twisting my body now during my normal course of living my life. I feel my confidence level continuing to grow.

I will keep it all going. Most of these small simple changes are soooo automatic now, from when I get out of bed in the morning, through the day, until I go to bed at night. All these small simple changes I have made over the past few months are really a part of me now. I will keep all this going bicep and triceps exercises, sitting leg lifts while at work in front of my computer, listening to positive personal and professional information on CDs and tapes during my commute, eating celery, doing crunches on the Ab machine in the morning and night, eating slower, snacking in between meals with the leftovers, drinking 5-7 bottles of water daily now, parking further away, stair walking, drinking green tea, going "manual" more, eating the multi-grain bread and wheat bread, doing 7-9 minutes of exercise when I get up, eating with my stomach not with my eyes, walking in the evening, replacing white flour products with wheat or multi-grains and cranking up the music with exercise in the morning and using that six-pack water carrying thingie to ensure I drink 5-7 bottles of water a day.

This week I will work on the eating side. During my commute I heard on a CD about blood sugar and something called a glycemic index for foods and how it relates to our blood sugar levels. The higher the index, the more it makes sugar spike in my system and makes me crash or drained afterwards. The speaker recommended eating foods or snacks with a lower index. Those types of food take longer to digest and their sugars are released throughout the body slower so I won't spike or crash. White bread was high, so I am good there. I already replaced that with wheat bread.

I will focus the bulk of my foods having a low index this week and see how that works for me.

Week 21 Small Simple Changes:

- ✓ Still Mad, but really feeling Good!
- ✓ Drank 3-5 Bottles of Water daily
- ✓ Parked Car further away at work and stores
- ✓ Looked at the Yellow Sticky note of my goal 4 times daily
- ✓ Ate slower and drank water before and during meals
- ✓ Ate leftovers and fruit in between meals
- ✓ Took Stairs to the 2nd Floor at work
- ✓ Drank Green Tea daily
- ✓ Went Manual
- ✓ Began simple exercises when I got out of bed to get the metabolism going
- ✓ Ate with my stomach not with my eyes - eat meals the size of your hand
- ✓ Took leisurely walks around the neighborhood
- ✓ Replaced all white flour products with wheat or multi/whole grains
- ✓ Added music to my morning exercises – cranked up exercises to 7-8 minutes
- ✓ Increased crunches by 10
- ✓ Replaced my "comfort food" cravings with celery and peanut butter and hummus
- ✓ Reviewed and reinforced my small simple changes
- ✓ Listened to positive personal and professional improvement tapes and CDs during my commute

- ✓ Filled up six-pack water carrying thingie with bottled water and finished each day
- ✓ Started sitting leg lifts while at work at my computer 5 reps, 2-3 times a day
- ✓ Reviewed small simple changes and reinforced all, especially those ones added in the past few weeks
- ✓ Incorporated some arm, biceps and triceps weight exercises into my morning exercise routine
- ✓ Started using that old Abdominal machine in the morning
- ✓ Started using that old Abdominal machine in the evening too
- ✓ Ate more foods with a lower glycemic index
- ✓ End of week weight: 210 pounds – lost 4 pounds

WEEK TWENTY-TWO

I am soooo pumped. Another 4 pounds gone. 4 must be a magic number for me. 210 pounds now. Getting into the single digits.

Consciously looking for foods with a lower glycemic index is fun. Sort of like investigating work. Once I found that chart, it was pretty easy to find foods that I like and have a low index.

Basically, lose the white flower stuff and eat more green stuff. I love broccoli anyway. Now I have a good reason to eat more of it. It really keeps the pipes flowing. I felt very light this week. No times of sluggishness at all.

Okay, recapping so far – daily checking of foods with lower a glycemic index, bicep and tricep exercises, sitting leg lifts while at work in front of my computer, listening to positive personal and professional information on CDs and tapes during my commute, eating celery, doing crunches on the Ab machine in the morning and night, eating slower, snacking in between meals with the leftovers, drinking 5-7 bottles of water daily, parking further away, stair walking, drinking green tea, going "manual" more, eating the multi-grain bread and wheat bread, doing 7-9 minutes of exercise when I get up, eating with my stomach not with my eyes, walking in the evening, replacing white flour products with wheat or multi-grains and cranking up the music with exercise in the morning and using that six-pack water carrying thingie to ensure I drink 5-7 bottles of water a day.

This week back to exercising – got to work on more muscles. I remember legs being the bigger muscles in the body. I am walking more.

I need to figure out some way to do weights with my legs at home. I know, I can do those sitting leg lifts in the morning and put my dumbbells on top of my knees to add more weight. I can also work on my leg muscles by flexing onto my toes while standing up and holding the dumbbells to my side. Yes, that is what I will do this week.

Week 22 Small Simple Changes:

- ✓ Still Mad, but really feeling Good!
- ✓ Drank 3-5 Bottles of Water daily
- ✓ Parked Car further away at work and stores
- ✓ Looked at the Yellow Sticky note of my goal 4 times daily
- ✓ Ate slower and drank water before and during meals
- ✓ Ate leftovers and fruit in between meals
- ✓ Took Stairs to the 2nd Floor at work
- ✓ Drank Green Tea daily
- ✓ Went Manual
- ✓ Began simple exercises when I got out of bed to get the metabolism going
- ✓ Ate with my stomach not with my eyes - eat meals the size of your hand
- ✓ Took leisurely walks around the neighborhood
- ✓ Replaced all white flour products with wheat or multi/whole grains
- ✓ Added music to my morning exercises – cranked up exercises to 7-8 minutes
- ✓ Increased crunches by 10
- ✓ Replaced my "comfort food" cravings with celery and peanut butter and hummus
- ✓ Reviewed and reinforced my small simple changes
- ✓ Listened to positive personal and professional improvement tapes and CDs during my commute

- ✓ Filled up six-pack water carrying thingie with bottled water and finished each day
- ✓ Started sitting leg lifts while at work at my computer 5 reps, 2-3 times a day
- ✓ Reviewed small simple changes and reinforced all, especially those ones added in the past few weeks
- ✓ Incorporated some arm, biceps and triceps weight exercises into my morning exercise routine
- ✓ Started using that old Abdominal machine in the morning
- ✓ Started using that old Abdominal machine in the evening too
- ✓ Ate more foods with a lower glycemic index
- ✓ Started leg exercises with light dumbbells at home
- ✓ End of week weight: 207 pounds – lost 3 pounds

WEEK TWENTY-THREE

3 more pounds gone. Down to 207 now. Almost there. I am so excited. I tailored as much of my clothes as possible, but I had to buy some new stuff. Some of the clothes I just could not tailor.

I went from over a 48 inch waist down to a 36 inch waist! That is over 1 foot of me lost – not height – width!!! It felt great buying clothes in the 30 inch range. It was exciting being able to wear a pants size that was less than my age finally!

Starting those leg exercises with light dumbbells at home is definitely building muscle that will burn fat at rest. Eating after I do those and walking in the evening seems to be burning fat off. I remember reading about how muscle not only burns fat at rest, but the after-burn effect of building muscles keeps going longer than with just plain cardio exercises.

Both are important for different reasons, but I like the fact building muscle not only burns fat when resting, but also right after the workout it has that after-burn effect longer than cardio exercise. Good piece of knowledge. Not sure how scientifically accurate it is, but hey, if my mind believes it, then my body will as well.

Leg exercises with light dumbbells, daily checking of foods with lower a glycemic index, biceps and triceps exercises, sitting leg lifts while at work in front of my computer and listening to positive personal and professional information on CDs and tapes during my commute is really having an impact on my body and mind.

Eating celery, doing crunches on the Ab machine in the morning and night, eating slower, snacking in between meals with the leftovers, drinking 5-7 bottles of water daily, parking further away, stair walking, drinking green tea, going "manual" more, eating the multi-grain bread and wheat bread is now soooo automatic.

Doing 7-9 minutes of exercise when I get up, eating with my stomach not with my eyes, walking in the evening, replacing white flour products with wheat or multi-grains and cranking up the music with exercise in the morning and using that six-pack water carrying thingie to ensure I drink 5-7 bottles of water a day is now part of my way of life.

This week I will focus on all of these. Especially looking for other ways to build natural muscles. I will not weigh myself this week since I am so close to my goal. I will skip weighing myself this week in anticipation of being less than 200 pounds in 2 short weeks. I have been averaging 2-3 pounds a week, I know I can blast through these last 7-8 pounds to get under 199 pounds soon, especially with this new found knowledge of the muscle-burning fat monster method.

Week 23 Small Simple Changes:

- ✓ Still Mad, but really feeling Good!
- ✓ Drank 3-5 Bottles of Water daily
- ✓ Parked Car further away at work and stores
- ✓ Looked at the Yellow Sticky note of my goal 4 times daily
- ✓ Ate slower and drank water before and during meals
- ✓ Ate leftovers and fruit in between meals
- ✓ Took Stairs to the 2nd Floor at work
- ✓ Drank Green Tea daily
- ✓ Went Manual
- ✓ Began simple exercises when I got out of bed to get the metabolism going
- ✓ Ate with my stomach not with my eyes - eat meals the size of your hand
- ✓ Took leisurely walks around the neighborhood
- ✓ Replaced all white flour products with wheat or multi/whole grains
- ✓ Added music to my morning exercises – cranked up exercises to 7-8 minutes
- ✓ Increased crunches by 10
- ✓ Replaced my "comfort food" cravings with celery and peanut butter and hummus
- ✓ Reviewed and reinforced my small simple changes
- ✓ Listened to positive personal and professional improvement tapes and CDs during my commute

- ✓ Filled up six-pack water carrying thingie with bottled water and finished each day
- ✓ Started sitting leg lifts while at work at my computer 5 reps, 2-3 times a day
- ✓ Reviewed small simple changes and reinforced all, especially those ones added in the past few weeks
- ✓ Incorporated some arm, biceps and triceps weight exercises into my morning exercise routine
- ✓ Started using that old Abdominal machine in the morning
- ✓ Started using that old Abdominal machine in the evening too
- ✓ Ate more foods with a lower glycemic index
- ✓ Did leg exercises with light dumbbells at home
- ✓ Kept focus on all my current Small Simple Changes and looked for other ways to increase use of my muscles to burn fat more efficiently
- ✓ End of week weight: did not weigh myself this week

WEEK TWENTY-FOUR

I know I lost more weight last week, but I don't want to focus on that this week. I feel SOOOOOOOOOOOOOO much better compared to when I think back from the beginning. I can't believe, just a few months ago, I could not tie my own shoes without huffing or puffing. I could not bend down to pick something up without doing some sort of strenuous gymnastics. I could not take a shower or go to the bathroom without difficulty.

Wow – what an INCREDIBLE improvement. Not only can effortlessly do all of these simple daily things, but I can do soooo much more. I have soooooo much more energy. My mind is clearer. I blast through my personal and professional 'to do" lists now.

My whole outlook on life is so much more positive now compared to several months ago. I noticed the ladies are actually checking me out now! That has not happened in a long time. Wow, I feel great.

Okay, since all these small simple changes have brought me this far, I will definitely keep them all going. Besides, it is hard to forget to do them – they are so automatic know. Putting the dumbbells near the bathroom is a super reminder to me to do my exercises in the morning.

Using that 6-pack water carrying thingie to remind me to bring and drink more water really works. I find myself going back in the house to get it when I did forget it – sort of like forgetting my car keys.

My buddy Tom played football in college and went to the Eagle camp to try out for pro ball. He is very athletic looking for a guy his age. Not a thin runner look, but a healthy respectable built look. I know he pumps iron at a gym. I will chat with him more about this. I know he doesn't spend hours every night there, because he has similar time commitments as I do with my job, family and community. I really like the idea of that muscle fat burner idea. I will chat more with him about what he does to keep in shape.

Week 24 Small Simple Changes:

- ✓ Still Mad, but really feeling Good!
- ✓ Drank 3-5 Bottles of Water daily
- ✓ Parked Car further away at work and stores
- ✓ Looked at the Yellow Sticky note of my goal 4 times daily
- ✓ Ate slower and drank water before and during meals
- ✓ Ate leftovers and fruit in between meals
- ✓ Took Stairs to the 2nd Floor at work
- ✓ Drank Green Tea daily
- ✓ Went Manual
- ✓ Began simple exercises when I got out of bed to get the metabolism going
- ✓ Ate with my stomach not with my eyes - eat meals the size of your hand
- ✓ Took leisurely walks around the neighborhood
- ✓ Replaced all white flour products with wheat or multi/whole grains
- ✓ Added music to my morning exercises – cranked up exercises to 7-8 minutes
- ✓ Increased crunches by 10
- ✓ Replaced my "comfort food" cravings with celery and peanut butter and hummus
- ✓ Reviewed and reinforced my small simple changes
- ✓ Listened to positive personal and professional improvement tapes and CDs during my commute

- ✓ Filled up six-pack water carrying thingie with bottled water and finished each day
- ✓ Started sitting leg lifts while at work at my computer 5 reps, 2-3 times a day
- ✓ Reviewed small simple changes and reinforced all, especially those ones added in the past few weeks
- ✓ Incorporated some arm, biceps and triceps weight exercises into my morning exercise routine
- ✓ Started using that old Abdominal machine in the morning
- ✓ Started using that old Abdominal machine in the evening too
- ✓ Ate more foods with a lower glycemic index
- ✓ Did leg exercises with light dumbbells at home
- ✓ Kept focus on all my current Small Simple Changes and looked for other ways to increase use of my muscles to burn fat more efficiently
- ✓ End of week weight: 198.5 – Initial GOAL Reached!!!!!!!!!!!!!!!!

WEEK TWENTY-FIVE

Victory Dance – The crowd roars – in this corner weighing in at a trim 198.5 pounds is Rich the Journey Kay!

Yeaaaaaaaaaaaaaaaaaaaaaaaaaaaaaaaaaaaaaahhhhhhhhhhhhhhhhhhhhh. I reached my initial goal of being less than 200 pounds within six months.

Goal Status: ACHIEVED!!!!!!!!!!!!

Now to continue on with the journey…

Week 25 Small Simple Changes:
- ✓ Feeling Really Good!
- ✓ Drank 6-8 Bottles of Water daily
- ✓ Parked Car further away at work and stores
- ✓ Looked at the Yellow Sticky note of my goal 4 times daily
- ✓ Ate slower and drank water before and during meals
- ✓ Ate leftovers and fruit in between meals

- ✓ Took Stairs to the 2nd Floor at work
- ✓ Drank Green Tea daily
- ✓ Went Manual
- ✓ Began simple exercises when I got out of bed to get the metabolism going
- ✓ Ate with my stomach not with my eyes - eat meals the size of your hand
- ✓ Took leisurely walks around the neighborhood
- ✓ Replaced all white flour products with wheat or multi/whole grains
- ✓ Added music to my morning exercises – cranked up exercises to 7-8 minutes
- ✓ Increased crunches by 10
- ✓ Replaced my "comfort food" cravings with celery and peanut butter and hummus
- ✓ Reviewed and reinforced my small simple changes
- ✓ Listened to positive personal and professional improvement tapes and CDs during my commute
- ✓ Filled up six-pack water carrying thingie with bottled water and finished each day
- ✓ Did sitting leg lifts while at work at my computer 5 reps, 2-3 times a day
- ✓ Reviewed small simple changes and reinforced all, especially those ones added in the past few weeks
- ✓ Continued arm, biceps and triceps weight exercises into my morning exercise routine
- ✓ Used that old Abdominal machine in the morning

✓ Used that old Abdominal machine in the evening too

✓ Ate more foods with a lower glycemic index

✓ Did leg exercises with light dumbbells at home

✓ Kept focus on all my current Small Simple Changes and looked for other ways to increase use of my muscles to burn fat more efficiently

✓ Talked to Tom about the next part of my journey

✓ Initial GOAL Reached!!!!!!!!!!!!!!!! Under 200 pounds – 198.5 pounds******

✓ Continuing on with the next part of the journey…

9

THE NEW BEGINNING

Congratulations again! You have finished the INITIAL reading of this book. This is not the end, but the beginning of a life long journey of continuously improving yourself. Getting back to the real you under all that extra weight you have been carrying around. A famous author, Ken Blanchard said "Feedback is the breakfast of champions." You are a Champion. You were created in the image of the creator. You have what it takes to reach your goals. I applaud you for taking these steps to the new you.

I encourage you to reread this book over and over again. We printed it in this small handy size to make it easier to carry around with you and refer to it often.

Now it's your turn. My recommendation to you is to decide you will make one small simple change in your eating and activity habits for the next 24 weeks and watch what happens.

Keep a journal to record your progress and review it often. You will be amazed at your progress over time.

Like what you read? I welcome your feedback. Email me at RichKay@RichKay.NET or call me at 866.250.7287 with your comments and success stories. Ask me about my availability to speak at your next event for your Group or Organization and Coaching services to reach a new level.

Godspeed and enjoy the journey,

Rich Kay
www.SmallSimpleChanges.com

10

A FINAL THOUGHT

When you introduce Small Simple Changes into your daily life they become new habits and will eventually move out and replace the old destructive habits.

I would like to think we all have sayings or quotes we like to hang onto and refer to often to inspire us and give us strength at various times in our life, especially challenging ones.

A quote I try to remind myself about often, especially when my motivation is low, is a verse from the Bible, New Testament, (NIV version): It is:

> "I can do all things through Christ, who strengthens me."
> Philippians 4:13

You CAN do ALL things, whether it is losing weight and getting back to the REAL you or whatever other challenges you encounter or goals you wish to achieve. You were created for success, endowed with seeds of greatness and assembled for achievement!

I wish you all the success in life that is awaiting you. Take action now to reach potential you have been blessed with.

ABOUT THE AUTHOR

Rich Kay has been where many adults struggle. At 277 pounds and just under six feet, he was obese and more than 100 pounds over his ideal weight. He had difficulties bending over to tie his shoes, getting out of bed in the morning and even going to the bathroom. He had countless medical issues from a fatty liver, sleep apnea, high cholesterol and depression to being a borderline diabetic. Rich had enough. He made a decision to win the battle of the bulge.

Within six months, he transformed into a vibrant, fit and energetic man on a mission.

He not only lost over 100 pounds, but also eliminated all the medical issues which were bringing him towards an early grave. Now his mission is to help others win their battle of the bulge once and for all and improve their quality of life through Small Simple Changes.

In his book, Small Simple Changes to Weight Loss and Weight Management, Rich Kay shares a series of dozens of Small Simple Changes he took over his 24-week journey to accomplish his goal. No fad diet, no starving yourself, no 2-hour gym workouts.

Read, see and hear his story for yourself and learn how to follow his successful method of shedding those unwanted pounds and keeping them off through his Small Simple Changes and begin your journey to Win the Battle of the Bulge once and for all!

Ask Rich about his availability to speak at your next event for your Group or Organization.

Call 866.250.7287 or email RichKay@RichKay.net to discuss how Rich can help you and your organization or go to www.SmallSimpleChanges.com to order more copies of his book.

LET'S STAY IN TOUCH:

1. Follow me on Twitter: RichKaySSC
2. Facebook: Small Simple Changes and join the group
3. Updates/motivation: go to www.SmallSimpleChanges.com
and register for email updates

———————————————

Need a different kind of Speaker to inspire, entertain and inform your church, community group, business or organization? Looking for a Coach to reach a new level?

Contact me at:
RichKay@RichKay.NET
866.250.7287
www.SmallSimpleChanges.com

SmallSimpleChanges.com
RichKay@RichKay.net
866.250.7287

ISBN 10: 1512019232
ISBN 13: 9781512019230

58348551R00057